How To Reverse Traction Alopecia Manual

A Step By Step Guide For Growing Back Your Hair

AUTHOR BREANNA RUTTER

TABLE OF CONTENTS

I0427853

INTRODUCTION TO
HOW TO REVERSE
TRACTION ALOPECIA MANUAL

"How To Reverse Traction Alopecia is a pocket guide that will help you to successfully grow back your hair through a variety of remedies and protective suggestions. There are many things that could have caused you to lose your hair such as; improper styling, hair care habits and even your choice of hair care products. Growing back your hair is a process that will include a wide array of solutions ranging from topical traction treatments, styling techniques, as well as the option to go the surgical route! Understanding how to grow back your hair will require a lot of patience and discipline on your end because the natural growth cycle of your hair has a lot to do with your recovery time.

This manual breaks down growing your hair in simple yet easy steps involving growth treatments, hair care regimens and styling techniques that lead to flourishing hair growth! The skills required to growing your hair back from Traction Alopecia are of a minimum skill level paired with a vast array of hair knowledge so that you can understand why you have to do certain things to your hair to maintain and encourage the health of it. This manual is here to thoroughly educate you about your hair loss in regards to alopecia as well as provide a multitude of solutions that will help grow back your hair and forever prevent this devastation from happening again!

Please enjoy this informative read and remain patient throughout the process as you are growing your hair back!"

Sincerely Breanna

1 HAIR GROWTH CYCLE

Understanding the life cycle of hair will give you the basic foundation of knowing how to diagnose a variety of problems you may encounter when growing healthy hair and achieving your goal lengths. Knowing the behavioral characteristics of hair growth will indicate whether or not your hair is growing, if the shedding you are experiencing is normal and also how quickly you can expect to see growth results. Knowing how long you should expect your traction alopecia to revert is crucial towards knowing if your growing efforts are really making difference!

Hair encounters three stages within its growth/life cycle. Each individual hair you are growing on your head can be present in different stages of its life cycle and because of that, you lose on average 80 to 100 strands of hair daily. Given that you have about 100,000 strands of hair on your head in total, don't be alarmed about shedding that many strands because this is a normal process that takes place. If you think about it, shedding makes up way less than 1% of the hair that you have on your scalp right now! Now let's discuss the life cycle of hair in further detail.

The Anagen Phase is the 1st phase of the hair life cycle as this is the growing phase because a new hair has begun growing. Since all of your hair is not in the Anagen Phase at once, it will take time before you will notice thickness because other hairs have to enter this phase as well. This phase lasts 2 to 6 years.

The Catagen Phase is the 2nd phase in which your hair is transitioning towards the Telogen phase. The hair is separating from your follicle (see definition guide) and moving upward towards your pore, or the surface of your scalp to fall out as shed hair. This phase lasts 1 to 2 weeks.

The Telogen Phase is the 3rd phase in which the hair is resting because the dermal papilla (see definition guide) separates from the follicle and then moves upward to begin growing a brand new hair. This phase lasts 2 to 4 months.

It is important that you completely understand the growth cycle of hair while recovering from traction alopecia damage so that you can gauge how long it should take for your hair to begin showing growth! The Telogen Phase and the Anagen Phase are the only two phases that allows you to see growth in hair. The time frame between these two phases are 2 months to 6 years. You should not have to wait 6 years to see your hair regrow because remember, all hair is not in the same phase of its life cycle at the same time!

The golden time frame to stick with when trying to grow your hair back from traction alopecia is no longer than 2 to 4 months time to notice growth. You should see growth in as little as 2 months and if you do not see growth, 4 months is the longest time you need to wait to see results of growth.

If you have remained consistent in trying a specific recommendation (recommendations to be suggested later) and you see no signs of growth within 2 to 4 months, go ahead and try another recommended hair growth solution until you find success with growing back your hair from traction alopecia!

2 UNDERSTANDING HAIR PH

Experiencing frizzy, dry and breaking hair is due large in part to keeping your hair PH balanced! Frizzy hair or damaged hair can ruin the look of many hairstyles with the most common being straight hair and then twists and braids. The reason why frizzy or damaged hair can be hard to beat is because the hair is not PH balanced! PH balance has a lot to do with the health and behavior of your hair especially when achieving certain looks. Your hair is left prone to breakage, and also has a hard time recovering from traction alopecia, if your hair is not in its ideal range of PH!

The PH scale is used to measure how acidic or alkaline a solution is and the scale ranges from 1 (acidic) to 14 (alkaline). Water has a PH of 7 (neutral) and is used to compare the acidity or alkalinity of a solution. The ideal PH range of hair is 4.5 to 5.5. Hair has an acidity of 4.5 to 5.5 and should remain this way especially if you want to achieve your most healthy hair. The reason why this is important when reversing traction alopecia is because when your hair is in contact with an acidic product, it will cause your cuticles (refer to definition guide) to flatten resulting in smooth & healthy moisturized strands of hair. When hair is in contact with an alkaline solution, the cuticles raise, the strands themselves swell (which can cause breakage) and this leads to frizzy, dry and ultimately, damaged hair!

To regrow your hair from traction alopecia, it's high priority to always keep your hair in the range of 4.5 to 5.5 and the best way to do this, is to make sure that you are using hair care products that are PH balanced. If you do not know the PH of your hair products, test your products with Litmus Strips. If you want products that are already PH balanced, I suggest HowToBlackHair.com referred hair care products specifically formulated for maintaining healthy hair.

3 TRACTION ALOPECIA FROM BRAIDS

Experiencing traction alopecia from braids is far from unheard of! Many women and men who experience traction alopecia from braids dismiss it by assuming that there edges have broken off badly or their hair just "grows slow" and that is why recovery is taking a significant amount of time. The average rate of hair growth is about 1/2 inch every month. A month alone of practicing good hairstyling habits and using quality hair care products should yield you some visible growth but for some, this is not the case.

Traction alopecia from braids begins after experiencing thinning and breakage from too tight braids. When your braids are braided too tightly, this causes your hairs to uproot themselves prematurely which in most cases, can leave you with a unflattering bald spot! Tight braids commonly show breakage or balding in the areas around the perimeter of your head (nape and edges) or at the very start of your braids. Also wearing braids that feel heavy, will cause traction alopecia as well. Keep in mind that your hairs are in different moments of its cycle so when breakage happens, it may take a while for your edges to grow in and then, for them to grow back to its original density.

Every time you braid your hair or allow someone else to braid your hair, your level of comfort should be a pain free install. Whoever said beauty is pain may have referenced to some other kind of cosmetic enhancement because painful installs cause traction alopecia!

If you want to learn how to do pain less beautiful braids on your own hair or for someone else, I highly recommend visiting HowToBlackHair.com to purchase a variety of braiding and hairstyling dvds!

4 TRACTION ALOPECIA FROM TWISTS

Experiencing traction alopecia from twists happens as well but not as frequent as braids. This may be due in part to the fact that the most popular hairstyles worn by African American women are individual braids and sew ins (with a braid base). Twists on the other hand can cause significant breakage as well if your hair is twisted too tightly! Some well-known hairstyles that consists of twists are Senegalese Twists, Havana Twists/Marley Twists, Flat Twists and so on. Specifically for natural hairstyles, some include styles like Two Strand Twists, Bantu Knots, and 3 Strand Twists for example.

Traction alopecia from twists begins after experiencing thinning and breakage from too tight twists, similarly to braids. Tight twists cause your hairs to uproot themselves prematurely and can leave you with a unflattering bald spot! Tight twists commonly show breakage or balding in the areas around the perimeter of your head (nape and edges) or at the very start of your twist. Heavy twists can also cause breakage along the length of your hair and traction alopecia especially when they are heavy. Remember, your hairs are in different moments of its cycle so when breakage happens, it may take a while for your hairs to grow in and then, for them to grow back to its original density as well.

Every time you twist your hair or allow someone else to twist your hair, your level of comfort should be a pain free install at all times. To avoid traction alopecia, avoid uncomfortable installs!

If you want to learn how to do pain less twists on your own hair or for someone else, I highly recommend visiting HowToBlackHair.com to purchase a variety of twisting and hairstyling dvds!

5 TRACTION ALOPECIA FROM WEAVES & EXTENSIONS

Experiencing traction alopecia from weaves and extensions are a constant threat for many who choose to wear these installs and this is not just affecting women of color. Women and men of all ethnicities are going for weaves and extensions as well for a change in look whether it be color or length.

Traction alopecia can happen easily while wearing weaves especially when your braids are too tight. It's perfectly okay to have firm braids but gripping the hair excessively while braiding does not ensure a neater braid nor does it extend the life of your braids! Many fail to realize that braids aggravate hair loss and if you do not braid in a firm but comfortable manner for your client or yourself, you will constantly battle with breakage and hair loss. Make it a priority for yourself and your client to assess whether or not the braids are causing pain. No one wants to remove their weave and take down their braids just to discover a bald or thinning area on their head!

Let's discuss sew ins for example, sew in installs are usually performed on a cornrow braid pattern base and this base can be constructed in a variety of ways such as the; Beehive, Double Beehive, Straight Backs, and Butterfly for example. The key to avoiding traction alopecia is to braid comfortably, protect your hair with a weaving net, and invest into quality hair extensions that do not cause a heavy feel.

If you want to learn how to do pain less weaves and extension hairstyles on your own hair or for someone else, I highly recommend visiting HowToBlackHair.com to purchase a variety of hairstyling dvds!

6 TRACTION HAIR GROWTH OILS

There are a multitude of hair care products available on the market that offer to repair a variety of hair problems many individuals suffer from today. Visit a local drug store to check out the beauty isle to inspect the hair care products. You will notice that most of the hair care products offer repair for problems such as split ends, fading color, flat thin hair and so on! The problem is that many products that promise hair growth are not actually formulated with ingredients that contribute to the growth of your hair. When reading the labels of many commercialized hair care products, you will notice that the most popular products are filled with ingredients such as; petrolatum, silicones, and sulfates! These are the worst ingredients known for hair because they cause buildup, breakage, and dry hair! To grow your hair back from traction alopecia, it is best to make sure that you are using ingredients that strengthen your hair from the inside out, encourage blood flow for optimal hair growth, and keep your hair PH balanced.

On the following pages are recipes for traction hair growth oils with a regimen that you can use in the comfort of your own home to help you grow your hair back. Please keep in mind the growth cycle of hair is in between 2 months to 6 years so give yourself 2 to 4 months, courtesy of the Anagen Phase, to truly see results of hair growth. If one recipe does not improve your hair as suggested, move onto another traction treatment after 4 months to find the solution that works for you!

Always perform a 24 hour patch test in a discrete area of your head. All recipes contribute to hair growth but some also offer the benefit of treating other hair problems as well!

TRACTION HAIR OIL RECIPES
(always 24 hour patch test for sensitivity)

Thoroughly mix any given solution in its own applicator bottle and store with a cap covering the spout to prevent the evaporation of your essential oil!

Rosemary Recipe
(For Growth)

- 5 drops Rosemary Essential Oil
- 1 oz/2 tbsp Virgin Cold Pressed Coconut Oil

Ylang Ylang Recipe
(For Strength)

- 5 drops Ylang Ylang Essential Oil
- 1 oz/2 tbsp Organic Sesame Oil

Peppermint Recipe
(For Increased Blood Flow)

- 5 drops Peppermint Essential Oil
- 1 oz/2 tbsp Organic Safflower Oil

Lavender Recipe
(For Inflammation)

- 5 drops Lavender Essential Oil
- 1 oz/2 tbsp Virgin Cold Pressed Olive Oil

Tea Tree Recipe
(For Dandruff/Itchiness)

- 5 drops Tea Tree Essential Oil
- 1 oz/2 tbsp Virgin Cold Pressed Grapeseed Oil

Jamaican Recipe
(For Growth + Strength)

- 1 oz/2 tbsp Organic Jamaican Black Castor Oil

TRACTION HAIR OIL APPLICATION + REGIMEN

THIS CAN BE DONE DAILY!

Step #1 Lubricate your fingers with your Traction Hair Oil Recipe of choice and GENTLY smooth oil onto your scalp and hair located in the area of your Traction Alopecia

Step #2 If possible, GENTLY two strand twist a 1/2 inch to 1 inch sections of hair in the damaged area to avoid additional manipulation from styling

If not possible, leave hair as is

DO NOT STYLE YOUR DAMAGED AREAS, APPLY TENSION OR APPLY ADDITIONAL PRODUCT WHATSOEVER!

7 NIGHT TIME ROUTINE

Your night time routine is vital for preserving the health of your hair and without this routine, you will constantly suffer from breakage and never recover from traction alopecia! Not only does handling your hair in a gentle manner dramatically decrease breakage, but so does your protective night time routine!

When performing your night time routine, it is very important that your damaged area of hair has been already prepped with your Traction Hair Oil Application. Before going to bed, you must always use the appropriate material to eliminate friction encountered throughout the night. The two choices of fabric that are best for protecting your hair throughout the night are Satin and Silk.

Satin is more affordable than silk, is the more flexible material and can be washed with ease. Satin does not cause friction on your hair and nor does Silk, but Satin causes more friction in comparison to Silk.

Silk is priced higher than satin, is not as flexible in comparison and has to be delicately hand washed or cleansed through a dry cleaning service. Silk does not cause friction on your hair or edges and nor does Satin, but Silk is superior in preventing friction than Satin is.

There are a few ways to protect your hair from friction with Silk or Satin material such as using a; Satin/Silk Pillowcase, Bonnet or Head Scarf. For growing back your hair from alopecia, it is preferred to sleep with a Bonnet or Scarf to prevent any friction throughout the night.

Following the suggested regimen allows you encourage growth by protecting your hair from additional friction.

NIGHT TIME ROUTINE

Step #1 Perform The Traction Hair Oil Application

Step #2 (For Satin/Silk Pillowcase)

Cover your bed pillow of choice with your case of choice. Double case your pillow if needed because of slippage.

Step #3 (For Satin/Silk Bonnet)

Wear a comfortable but secure bonnet that covers all of your hair If the bonnet feels tight or too loose to stay secure, seek another bonnet or protection of choice.

Step #4 (For Satin/Silk Head Scarf)

Secure your scarf around your head in a way that covers all of your hair including your edges.

IMPORTANT Alternate the tied knot of your head scarf in a new position on your hairline every night. Constantly knotting the scarf at the same point along your hairline can lead to thinning!

8 SAFE HAIRSTYLING OPTIONS

You must carefully consider your choice of extensions and how much manipulation is required to complete a look you desire as well as preserve the health of your area of alopecia. Often times, hairstyling is the culprit to many who lost the their hair to traction alopecia! Below are lists of some of the worst and best hairstyles to wear to help you grow back your affected area of hair. One important thing to remember is that the more hairs contained within a given braid or twist, the stronger your hair will be within the braid or twist.

WORST HAIRSTYLES FOR TRACTION ALOPECIA
Micro Braids – small braids cause breakage easily
Kinky Twist (small) – small twists cause breakage easily
Ponytail Sew In – exposed hair edges/nape can break easily
Partial Sew In – leave out experiences breakage easily
Yarn Braids – yarn is too heavy for unhealthy hair
Yarn Wraps – yarn is too heavy for unhealthy hair
U-Part/L-Part Wig – leave out experiences breakage easily
Quick Weave – unhealthy hair will tear from glue removal

BEST HAIRSTYLES FOR TRACTION ALOPECIA
Jumbo Individual Braids – large braids decrease breakage
Kinky Twists (large) – large twists decrease breakage
Net Weave Full Sew In – tension is on net instead of edges
Invisible Part Sew In – smooth edges instead when finished

Even though there are more choices than listed here for best hairstyles, it's most important to leave the damaged hair or alopecia area without additional hair products or tensions from weaves, extensions, braids or twists. If your edges are damaged, slick down the edges of your hair while damp with a molding strip instead of applying tension from styles or using additional products like hair gel.

9 CHEMICAL RELAXERS

Some of those who are reading this manual may have relaxed hair and relaxing your hair can greatly stunt your growth while recovering from traction alopecia! When relaxing, it's good practice to always use chemical relaxers with caution and stretch your touch ups as far apart from one another as possible because hair loss is always a risk when chemically relaxing your hair.

Chemical relaxers and their dangers are heavily discussed in my book, The Relaxed Hair Bible: The 10 Commandments of Long Healthy Relaxed Hair so if you want to learn concentrated information on their usage, regimens, hair care treatments and more, refer to that book for detailed information. Furthermore, it's important to understand the dangers of using chemical relaxers when trying to recover from alopecia. Since this manual is focused on re-growing your hair from this kind of hair loss, doing everything possible to grow back healthy hair is priority and that is why it is suggested to stop chemically relaxing your hair until you recover!

This may be hard advice to follow for those who chose to chemically relax their hair but if you postpone your touch ups until you have recovered from traction alopecia, this will guarantee you the most success with your hair growth. As discussed in the Relaxed Hair Bible, chemical relaxers are highly alkaline and they disintegrate (or break down) your hairs to the point of straightness. When a relaxer is left on for too long or too high of strength is used, this can cause your hair to melt or worse, cause chemical burns! Because relaxers disrupt the PH of your hair and scalp, you have to resist using relaxers until you recover from traction alopecia. Once your hair is healthy, you can then proceed to relax your hair again!

10 SURGICAL RESTORATION

Surgical hair restoration is suggested for those who have truly given every Traction Hair Growth Oil, and a change in diet (Dieting For Hair Growth Manual) a fair and independent chance. Before going under the knife, give each recommended remedy its chance to produce results within a time frame of 2 to 4 months.

A natural approach to growing your hair back from alopecia offers a lower price point than surgery but, it is still completely up to you and understandable to seek surgical hair restoration and there are two options to consider if you want to surgically restore your hair permanently!

FUE Hair Transplant: Follicular Unit Extraction
FUT Hair Transplant: Follicular Unit Transplant

The FUE transplant requires individual follicles to be extracted from your scalp after injecting a local anesthesia to the preferred area of extraction. This procedure involves implanting your individual follicles throughout your thinning or bald area of scalp. A positive to this procedure is that it does not require staples/stiches, leaves behind no scars, and requires little recovery time. The negative is that it can take multiple procedures to achieve your desired result of density.

The FUT transplant requires a thin patch of scalp removed preferably from the back of your head after injecting a local anesthesia. This procedure involves dissecting your scalp into patches of 2 to 4 follicle units that will be inserted into your desired scalp area. The positive of this procedure is that it can be done in one session. The negative is that it can leave behind a scar, requires staples/stiches and has a lengthy recovery time.

AFTERWORDS

"This manual of course was made in mind for those who desire step by step help with growing their hair back from Traction Alopecia. As you may have read throughout these chapters, this manual is condensed with priceless information for helping you successfully recover from the hair damage you have unfortunately experienced. You may have chosen to read this guide because you support my work, you were looking for information on growing your hair back from Traction Alopecia, or you were looking for this information to help a loved one.

Personally, I have never had problems with traction alopecia or damaged edges but I have had my issues with dry hair and breaking ends. But what is to be noted is that it is perfectly fine if you do not have the same density of hair throughout your entire head. The edges of my hair and the nape are a little bit finer and at a lower density than the rest of my hair. This does not bother me and it does not mean that my hair is thinning or damaged. I have never had problems with breakage or thinning on my edges because I take great care of my hair. What has been golden for retaining length on my edges and nape hairs, has been from two strand twisting medium to small sections of hair to limit the amount of manipulation while handling the rest of my hair. I'm constantly overwhelmed by women and men who suffer with Traction Alopecia and have tried so desperately fix this problem and reaching out to me has been their last hope for recovery. This manual is inspired by those individuals because I am too passionate about hair not to help you especially when you need it the most!

I hope that you thoroughly enjoyed this read, it was a pleasure of mine to write this for your knowledge and enjoyment." Sincerely, Breanna

ADDITIONAL RESOURCES

The Official Website: www.Howtoblackhair.com

The Online Store: www.HowtoblackhairStore.com

Free Subscription Email: http://eepurl.com/FZs5b

For Additional Hair Questions

YourHairQuestions@Gmail.com

Black Hair Styling Tutorials

BlackWomenHair YouTube Channel

www.Youtube.com/BlackWomenHair

HowToBlackHair YouTube Channel

www.Youtube.com/HowToBlackHair

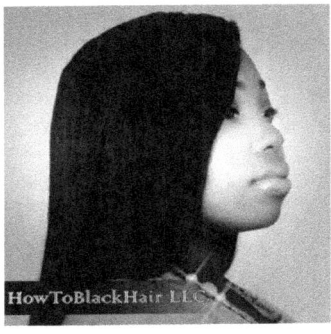

The Natural Hair Bible

The 10 Commandments of Black Hair Care

www.HowToBlackHair.com

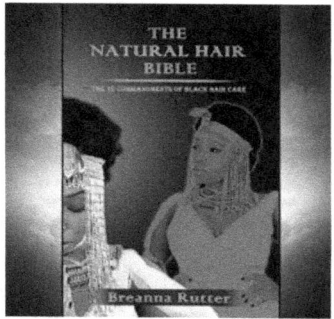

The Relaxed Hair Bible

The 10 Commandments of Long Healthy Relaxed Hair

www.HowToBlackHair.com

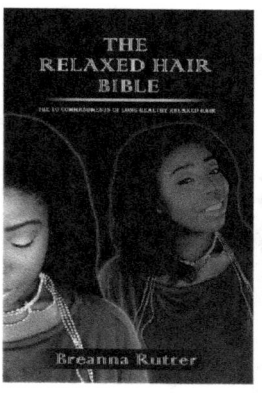

Black Hair Styling DVDs (Over 20+ Hairstyles)

www.HowToBlackHair.com

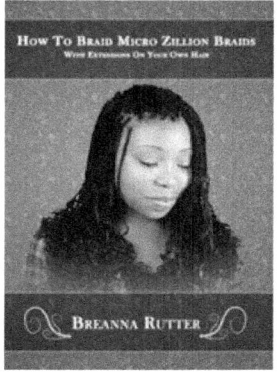 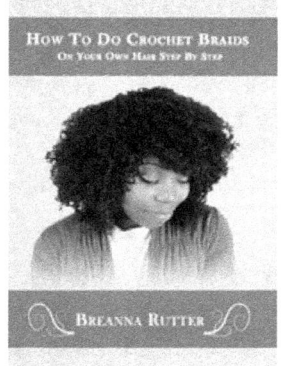

DEFINITION GUIDE

Anagen Phase: *the growth phase of the hair cycle*

Catagen Phase: *the transitioning phase of the hair cycle*

Cuticles: *a naturally protecting shield (arranged like shingles to the roof of a home) outside of your hair strands*

Dermal Papilla: *a raised dermis located underneath the root of your follicle that houses the blood supply*

Follicle: *an individual strand of hair*

FUE Hair Transplant: *Follicular Unit Extraction*

FUT Hair Transplant: *Follicular Unit Transplant*

Telogen Phase: *the rest phase of the hair cycle*

Traction Alopecia: *gradual hair loss usually caused by a pulling force on your hair from hair styling*

INDEX

TREATMENTS: *5, 12 & 18*
TWISTS: *8, 10, 14, 17 & 20*
WEAVES: *11 & 17*

HOW TO BLACK HAIR LLC.
WRITTEN BY BREANNA RUTTER
BOOK DESIGNED BY BREANNA RUTTER
COVER DESIGNED BY JARED RUTTER
ALL RIGHTS RESERVED.
VISIT WWW.HOWTOBLACKHAIR.COM

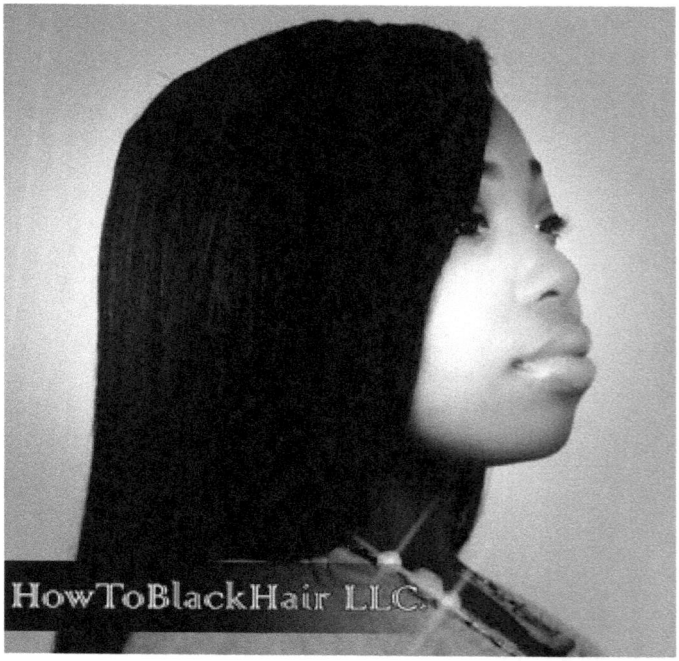

DISCLAIMER: All suggestions, techniques & advice given are for informational purposes only & should be used at your discretion & best judgment. I highly recommend conducting strand tests when trying or using new products, hair appliances & product mixes. I am not responsible or liable for adverse or undesirable affects including hair loss, hair breakage or other hair/scalp/skin/body damage as a direct or indirect result of the suggestions, tips, techniques &/or advice given.